PANCREATITIS COOKBOOK AND MEAL PLAN

"Pancreatitis Plates: *Nourishing Recipes and Meal Plans for a Healthy Digestive System"*

MATILDA TRUST

INTRODUCTION

    Causes of Pancreatitis

    Types of Pancreatitis

    The Role of Nutrition

    Meal Planning

    The Purpose of the Cookbook

CHAPTER 1

    Understanding Pancreatitis

    Importance Of A Pancreatitis-Friendly Diet

    Some specific foods that are beneficial for those with pancreatitis include

    How To Use This Book

CHAPTER 2

    Pancreatitis Cookbook

    A. Breakfast Recipes

    B. Snacks and Appetizers

    C. Soups and Salads

    D. Main Dishes

    E. Sides and Vegetables

    F. Desserts and Sweets

CHAPTER 3

    Pancreatitis Meal Plan

    A. 7-Day Pancreatitis Meal Plan

B. Grocery Shopping List

C. Meal Planning Tips and Tricks

CHAPTER 4

Bonus Resources

A. Pancreatitis-Friendly Ingredients Guide

B. Frequently Asked Questions (FAQs)

C. Tools and Equipment Recommended

CONCLUSION

INTRODUCTION

Pancreatitis cookbook and meal plan aim to provide essential information to readers regarding pancreatitis, its symptoms, causes, and effects on the body. It also outlines the importance of proper nutrition for individuals with pancreatitis and the role of diet in handling the ailment.

This helps readers to understand why nutrition is critical in managing the condition.

Causes of Pancreatitis: It is important to explain the potential causes of pancreatitis, including alcohol abuse, gallstones, certain medications, and genetics.

Types of Pancreatitis: There are two types of pancreatitis: acute and chronic. The introduction explains the differences between these two types and the long-term effects of chronic pancreatitis.

The Role of Nutrition: Nutrition is essential for individuals with pancreatitis, as it can help manage symptoms and improve quality of life. The introduction should explain the importance of proper nutrition and how it can benefit individuals with pancreatitis.

Meal Planning: The introduction provides an overview of meal planning for individuals with pancreatitis. This includes information on the types of foods to eat and avoid, meal timing, and portion control.

The Purpose of the Cookbook: This explains the purpose of the cookbook and how it can help individuals with pancreatitis. It also provides an overview of what the cookbook contains, such as easy-to-follow recipes, nutritional information, and tips for meal planning.

Proper nutrition can help manage symptoms and improve quality of life.

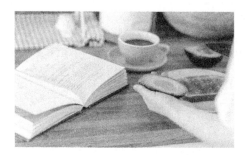

CHAPTER 1

Understanding

Pancreatitis

Pancreatitis is a condition that occurs when the pancreas, a gland located behind the stomach, becomes inflamed. The inflammation can be acute, which means it develops suddenly and lasts for a short time, or chronic, which means it develops slowly and lasts for a long time.

The causes of pancreatitis can vary, but the most common causes are alcohol abuse and gallstones. Other potential causes include high levels of triglycerides in the blood, certain medications, infections, genetic mutations, and trauma to the pancreas.

Symptoms of pancreatitis can include severe abdominal pain, nausea and vomiting, fever, rapid heartbeat, and dehydration. In severe cases, pancreatitis can lead to complications such as pancreatic necrosis, which is the death of pancreatic tissue, and organ failure.

Diagnosis of pancreatitis typically involves a physical exam, blood tests, imaging tests such as ultrasound or CT scan, and sometimes a biopsy of the pancreas. Treatment may involve hospitalization, fasting to rest the pancreas, pain medication, and intravenous fluids. In severe cases, surgery may be necessary to remove damaged tissue or treat complications.

Prevention of pancreatitis involves avoiding excessive alcohol consumption, maintaining a healthy weight, and treating underlying conditions such as high triglycerides or gallstones. For individuals with chronic pancreatitis, management may involve dietary changes and taking pancreatic enzyme supplements to aid in digestion.

Importance Of A Pancreatitis-Friendly Diet

Pancreatitis is a condition that occurs when the pancreas, an organ located in the abdomen, becomes inflamed. This inflammation can cause a variety of symptoms, including abdominal pain, nausea, vomiting, and fever. Pancreatitis can be acute or chronic, and can be caused by a number of factors, including alcohol consumption, gallstones, and certain medications.

One of the most important factors in managing pancreatitis is following a pancreatitis-friendly diet. A pancreatitis-friendly diet is one that is low in fat and high in nutrients, such as fruits, vegetables, whole grains, and lean protein. This type of diet can help to reduce inflammation in the pancreas and improve digestive function.

Some specific foods that are beneficial for those with pancreatitis include:

Fruits and vegetables: These foods are high in fiber and antioxidants, which can help to reduce inflammation and promote healthy digestion. Some good options include apples, berries, spinach, and broccoli.

Whole grains: Whole grains are a good source of fiber and complex carbohydrates, which can help to regulate blood sugar levels and promote satiety. Some good options include brown rice, quinoa, and whole wheat bread.

Lean protein: Protein is important for building and repairing tissue, but it's important to choose lean sources of protein, such as chicken, fish, and tofu. Fatty meats can be hard to digest and can exacerbate pancreatitis symptoms.

Healthy fats: While it's important to limit fat intake overall, it's still important to consume some healthy fats, such as those found in nuts, seeds, and avocado. These fats can help to reduce inflammation and support healthy digestion.

On the other hand, there are also some foods that should be avoided or limited when following a pancreatitis-friendly diet. These include:

Fatty or fried foods: These types of foods can be hard to digest and can exacerbate inflammation in the pancreas. Some examples include fried chicken, French fries, and pizza.

Sugary foods: Consuming too much sugar can disrupt blood sugar levels and exacerbate inflammation. Some examples include candy, soda, and baked goods.

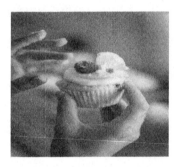

Alcohol: Alcohol can be a major contributor to pancreatitis, and should be avoided altogether if possible.

In addition to following a pancreatitis-friendly diet, it's also important to stay hydrated and to avoid smoking, as smoking can exacerbate inflammation in the pancreas. It's also important to work closely with a healthcare provider to manage pancreatitis symptoms and to ensure that any underlying causes of pancreatitis are addressed.

How To Use This Book

Consult with your healthcare provider: Before starting any new meal plan, it's important to talk to your healthcare provider, especially if you have pancreatitis. Your healthcare provider can help you determine what types of foods you should include and exclude from your diet.

Follow the recipes and meal plan as closely as possible: When using a cookbook or meal plan, it's important to follow the recipes and meal plan as closely as possible. This ensures that you are getting the right balance of nutrients and avoiding any foods that may exacerbate your pancreatitis.

Pay attention to portion sizes: Even if a recipe is made with pancreatitis-friendly ingredients, it's important to pay attention to portion sizes. Eating too much of any food can cause discomfort or worsen your symptoms.

Experiment with substitutions: If you find that a recipe or ingredient doesn't work for you, experiment with substitutions. For example, if a recipe calls for garlic and onions, but you find that they trigger your symptoms, you can try substituting with other herbs and spices.

Keep a food diary: Keeping a food diary can help you track what you eat and how it affects your pancreatitis symptoms. This information can be helpful for both you and your healthcare provider in managing your condition.

Don't hesitate to ask for help: If you're having trouble with a recipe or meal plan, don't hesitate to ask for help. There are many resources available, including online support groups and dietitians who specialize in pancreatitis.

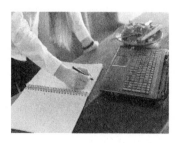

CHAPTER 2

Pancreatitis Cookbook

People with pancreatitis often experience symptoms such as abdominal pain, nausea, vomiting, and diarrhea.

A pancreatitis cookbook is a collection of recipes that are specifically designed for people with pancreatitis. These recipes are usually low in fat and easy to digest, which can help reduce symptoms and improve overall health.

Here are some key features of a pancreatitis cookbook:

Low-fat recipes: Since high-fat foods can exacerbate symptoms of pancreatitis, a pancreatitis cookbook will typically focus on recipes that are low in fat. This means that recipes may use lean meats, such as chicken or turkey, and avoid high-fat ingredients like butter or cream.

Easy-to-digest recipes: Digestive issues are common with pancreatitis, so a cookbook may include recipes that are easy to digest. This can involve cooking techniques that are gentle on the stomach, such as poaching or steaming, and avoiding ingredients that are difficult to digest, such as beans or spicy foods.

Nutrient-dense ingredients: A pancreatitis cookbook will often feature recipes that are high in nutrients, such as fruits and vegetables, to help support overall health. The cookbook may also include tips on how to increase nutrient intake while keeping fat intake low.

Meal planning and preparation tips: A pancreatitis cookbook may provide guidance on how to plan meals that are appropriate for the condition, as well as tips on how to prepare food in a way that is easy on the stomach. This can include suggestions for meal timing, portion control, and cooking techniques.

Supportive information: In addition to recipes, a pancreatitis cookbook may also include supportive information on the condition. This can include advice on managing symptoms, tips for navigating social situations while following a low-fat diet, and suggestions for working with a healthcare provider to manage the condition.

In summary, a pancreatitis cookbook is a resource that provides recipes, meal planning guidance, and supportive information for people with pancreatitis. By focusing on low-fat, easy-to-digest recipes that are high in nutrients, a pancreatitis cookbook can help people manage their symptoms and improve their overall health.

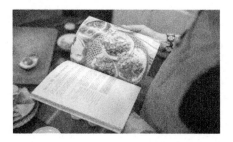

A. Breakfast Recipes

Breakfast recipes suitable for a pancreatitis cookbook meal plan:

Oatmeal: Oatmeal is a great breakfast option for those with pancreatitis because it is low in fat and high in fiber. You can prepare it with water or skim milk and add some fruit for sweetness.

Scrambled Eggs: Eggs are a good source of protein and can be prepared in a low-fat manner by using cooking spray instead of butter or oil. You can add some vegetables like spinach or bell peppers for extra nutrition.

Yogurt Parfait: Yogurt is a good source of protein and calcium, but make sure to choose a low-fat or non-fat variety. Layer the yogurt with some low-fat granola and fresh berries for a nutritious and delicious breakfast.

Smoothies: Smoothies are an excellent way to get a variety of nutrients in one meal. You can make a low-fat smoothie by using skim milk or yogurt as the base, and adding in some fruits and vegetables.

Toast with Peanut Butter: Peanut butter is a good source of protein and healthy fats, but it should be consumed in moderation due to its calorie density. Choose whole-grain bread and spread a thin layer of peanut butter on top.

Cottage Cheese with Fruit: Cottage cheese is a good source of protein and calcium, but make sure to choose a low-fat variety. Top it with some fresh fruit like strawberries or blueberries for a delicious and nutritious breakfast.

Breakfast Burrito: You can make a low-fat breakfast burrito by using a whole-grain tortilla, scrambled eggs, and some vegetables like bell peppers and onions. Top it with a small amount of salsa for extra flavor.

Remember to always consult with a healthcare professional or a registered dietitian to create a personalized meal plan that meets your individual needs and preferences.

B. Snacks and Appetizers

Hummus and Vegetables: Hummus is a good source of protein and healthy fats, and can be paired with a variety of vegetables such as carrot sticks, cucumber slices, and cherry tomatoes.

Low-Fat Cheese and Crackers: Choose a low-fat cheese such as string cheese or reduced-fat cheddar, and pair it with whole-grain crackers for a satisfying snack.

Fruit and Yogurt: Choose a low-fat or non-fat yogurt and pair it with fresh fruit such as apple slices, strawberries, or grapes for a healthy and refreshing snack.

Baked Sweet Potato Fries: Sweet potatoes are a good source of fiber and vitamins, and can be sliced into wedges and baked in the oven for a low-fat and tasty snack.

Edamame: Edamame is a good source of protein and can be steamed and lightly salted for a healthy and satisfying snack.

Vegetable Soup: Vegetable soup can be a nutritious and filling snack, especially when made with low-sodium broth and a variety of vegetables such as carrots, celery, and green beans.

Rice Cakes with Peanut Butter: Rice cakes are a low-fat and crunchy snack that can be topped with a thin layer of peanut butter for extra protein and flavor.

Remember to always consult with a healthcare professional or a registered dietitian to create a personalized meal plan that meets your individual needs and preferences. Additionally, it is important to limit or avoid high-fat or high-sugar snacks and processed foods that may exacerbate pancreatitis symptoms.

C. Soups and Salads

When creating a cookbook meal plan for someone with pancreatitis, it's important to focus on foods that are easy to digest and gentle on the pancreas.

Soups and salads that would be appropriate for a pancreatitis cookbook meal plan:

Soups:

Broth-based soups are a good option, as they are easy to digest and low in fat.

Avoid cream-based soups, as they are higher in fat and can be harder to digest.

Vegetable soups are a good choice, as they are high in nutrients and fiber.

Consider adding some lean protein, such as chicken or tofu, to your soups for added nutrition.

Avoid adding any spicy or acidic ingredients, as they can irritate the pancreas.

Salads:

Stick to simple salads with few ingredients to avoid overwhelming the digestive system.

Choose fresh, nutrient-dense ingredients such as leafy greens, vegetables, and lean proteins.

Avoid high-fat dressings such as creamy or oil-based dressings.

Consider using vinaigrette made with apple cider vinegar or lemon juice, which can help with digestion.

Avoid adding any spicy or acidic ingredients, as they can irritate the pancreas.

Overall, when creating a cookbook meal plan for pancreatitis, it's important to focus on foods that are easy to digest and low in fat. Soups and salads can be a great way to get in plenty of nutrients while still being gentle on the pancreas.

D. Main Dishes

When creating a meal plan for someone with pancreatitis, it's important to focus on foods that are gentle on the digestive system and low in fat.

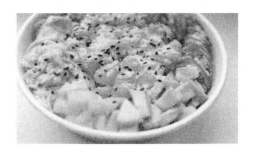

Some concepts below for main dishes:

Baked Salmon: Salmon is a great source of protein and healthy omega-3 fatty acids. Bake it in the oven with some lemon juice, herbs, and a little bit of olive oil.

Turkey Meatballs: Ground turkey is a lean source of protein. Mix it with some breadcrumbs, egg, and herbs and bake in the oven. Serve with a low-fat tomato sauce.

Lentil Soup: Lentils are a great source of plant-based protein and fiber. Make a lentil soup with low-sodium broth, carrots, celery, and onions. Add some spices for flavor.

Quinoa Salad: Quinoa is a nutritious grain that is easy to digest. Mix cooked quinoa with chopped vegetables like cucumbers, tomatoes, and bell peppers. Add a low-fat dressing.

Chicken Stir Fry: Use boneless, skinless chicken breast and stir-fry it with some vegetables like broccoli, bell peppers, and carrots. Use a low-fat stir-fry sauce.

Remember to avoid high-fat meats, fried foods, and creamy sauces. Stick to lean protein, vegetables, and whole grains.

E. Sides and Vegetables

When it comes to creating a meal plan for someone with pancreatitis, it is important to choose sides and vegetables that are gentle on the digestive system and do not exacerbate inflammation.

Selecting sides and vegetables for a pancreatitis cookbook meal plan:

Choose non-starchy vegetables: Vegetables such as leafy greens, broccoli, cauliflower, zucchini, and cucumber are low in carbohydrates and gentle on the digestive system.

Avoid high-fat sides: Avoid sides that are high in fat, such as creamed vegetables, fried foods, and creamy dips. Instead, choose sides that are baked, roasted, or steamed.

Incorporate whole grains: Whole grains such as brown rice, quinoa, and whole-wheat pasta are good sources of fiber and can be a healthy addition to the meal plan.

Limit canned vegetables: Canned vegetables may contain added salt and preservatives, which can be harmful for people with pancreatitis. Choose fresh or frozen vegetables instead.

Avoid spicy vegetables: Spicy vegetables such as hot peppers and onions can irritate the digestive system and increase inflammation. Instead, choose mild vegetables such as carrots, sweet potatoes, and butternut squash.

Incorporate herbs and spices: Use herbs and spices such as ginger, turmeric, and cinnamon to add flavor to vegetables without adding salt or fat.

Watch out for high-sugar sides: Sides that are high in sugar, such as sweetened fruit salads or candied yams can lead to blood sugar spikes and inflammation. Choose sides that are naturally sweet, such as roasted sweet potatoes or baked apples.

Overall, it is important to choose sides and vegetables that are gentle on the digestive system, low in fat and sugar, and rich in nutrients. With a little creativity, you can create delicious and healthy side dishes that are safe for people with pancreatitis.

F. Desserts and Sweets

When it comes to desserts and sweets for a pancreatitis cookbook meal plan, there are a few key things to keep in mind. First and foremost, it's important to choose options that are low in fat and sugar, as both of these can exacerbate pancreatitis symptoms.

Some ideas for desserts and sweets that is pancreatitis-friendly:

Opt for fruit-based desserts: Fresh fruit, fruit salad, or fruit compote are all excellent choices for a pancreatitis meal plan. They're low in fat and sugar, and they provide plenty of vitamins and fiber.

Stick with low-fat dairy products: If you're craving something creamy, opt for low-fat yogurt, pudding, or custard. Avoid full-fat dairy products, as these can be too rich for a pancreatitis diet.

Use alternative sweeteners: Instead of sugar, consider using alternative sweeteners like stevia, honey, or maple syrup. These options are less likely to cause a spike in blood sugar levels, which can be harmful for people with pancreatitis.

Avoid fried or greasy desserts: Fried foods are a no-go for pancreatitis patients, as they can be difficult to digest and may exacerbate symptoms. Stick with baked or grilled options instead.

Watch your portion sizes: Even if you're choosing pancreatitis-friendly desserts, it's important to be mindful of your portion sizes. Overeating can put strain on your pancreas and worsen symptoms.

Experiment with flavors: Don't be afraid to try new flavor combinations or ingredients in your desserts. For example, adding a dash of cinnamon to your fruit salad or drizzling balsamic vinegar over fresh berries can add an unexpected twist to your sweet treats.

Overall, desserts and sweets can still be a part of a pancreatitis meal plan, as long as they're chosen carefully and consumed in moderation.

CHAPTER 3

Pancreatitis Meal Plan

Pancreatitis is a condition that causes inflammation in the pancreas, which can lead to a range of digestive issues. Following a proper diet can be helpful in managing the symptoms of pancreatitis and promoting healing.

Pancreatitis meal plan:

Avoid alcohol: Alcohol is one of the leading causes of pancreatitis. Therefore, it's crucial to avoid alcoholic beverages if you have this condition.

Limit fat intake: A low-fat diet is essential for pancreatitis. Eating foods high in fat can trigger inflammation and cause pain. It's recommended to consume no more than 30 grams of fat per day, with most of the fat coming from healthy sources such as nuts, seeds, and fish.

Choose lean protein: Lean protein sources such as chicken, turkey, fish, and tofu are easier to digest and less likely to cause inflammation than fatty meats. It's also essential to cook the protein well and avoid using added fats.

Eat small meals frequently: Eating small, frequent meals throughout the day is beneficial for pancreatitis. It helps to keep the digestive system working efficiently and reduces the strain on the pancreas.

Include high-fiber foods: Foods high in fiber, such as fruits, vegetables, whole grains, and legumes, are beneficial for pancreatitis. They help to regulate digestion and promote healing in the digestive tract.

Stay hydrated: Drinking enough water is essential for pancreatitis. It helps to flush out toxins from the body and keeps the digestive system working efficiently.

Avoid spicy foods: Spicy foods can cause irritation and inflammation in the pancreas, so it's best to avoid them.

Consult a registered dietitian: Consulting a registered dietitian can be beneficial for developing a customized meal plan for pancreatitis based on individual needs and preferences.

By following a pancreatitis meal plan, individuals can manage their symptoms, promote healing in the digestive tract, and prevent future flare-ups.

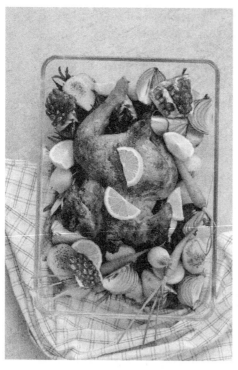

1 SPICY FOOD

A. 7-Day Pancreatitis Meal Plan

DAY 1

Avoid high-fat foods: Pancreatitis is a condition where the pancreas becomes inflamed, which can cause digestive problems. High-fat foods can exacerbate these symptoms and should be avoided. This includes foods like fried foods, fatty meats, dairy products, and processed foods.

DAY 2

Focus on lean proteins: Lean proteins like chicken, fish, turkey, and tofu are easier for the pancreas to digest and can provide important nutrients. Avoid red meats and fatty cuts of poultry.

DAY 3

Choose low-glycemic index carbohydrates: Carbohydrates that are high in sugar or refined flour can spike blood sugar levels, which can put additional strain on the pancreas. Choose whole grains, fruits, and vegetables that are low on the glycemic index.

DAY 4

Incorporate healthy fats: While it's important to avoid high-fat foods, it's also important to incorporate healthy fats into the diet. These can come from sources like nuts, seeds, avocados, and olive oil.

DAY 5

Stay hydrated: Drinking plenty of water can help flush toxins from the body and support healthy digestion. Avoid sugary drinks and limit caffeine and alcohol, which can irritate the pancreas.

DAY 6

Eat small, frequent meals: Eating smaller meals more frequently throughout the day can be easier on the pancreas than large meals. Aim for 5-6 smaller meals per day rather than 3 large meals.

Work with a healthcare provider or dietitian: Pancreatitis can be a serious condition and it's important to work with a healthcare provider or registered dietitian to create an individualized meal plan that meets your specific needs. They can help you identify trigger foods, adjust your diet as needed, and monitor your progress.

B. Grocery Shopping List

Avoid high-fat foods: People with pancreatitis should avoid foods that are high in fat because the pancreas is responsible for producing enzymes that help digest fats. Eating a lot of fat can put a strain on the pancreas and cause pain and inflammation.

Choose lean proteins: Instead of red meat, which is high in fat, choose lean proteins such as chicken, turkey, fish, and tofu. These are easier for the pancreas to digest and are less likely to cause inflammation.

Incorporate low-fiber fruits and vegetables: Raw vegetables and fruits with high fiber content can be difficult to digest for people with pancreatitis. Choose low-fiber options like cooked or canned vegetables and fruits like bananas, melons, and peaches.

Include complex carbohydrates: Choose complex carbohydrates like whole grains, beans, and lentils that are low in fat and high in fiber. These can help you feel full and satisfied while also being gentle on your pancreas.

Avoid alcohol and caffeine: Alcohol and caffeine can stimulate the pancreas and cause pain and inflammation. It's best to avoid these altogether or consume them in moderation.

Choose low-fat dairy products: Dairy products can be a good source of calcium, but they can also be high in fat. Choose low-fat options like skim milk, low-fat yogurt, and reduced-fat cheese.

Use healthy oils: When cooking, use healthy oils like olive oil or canola oil instead of butter or other high-fat oils.

Based on these guidelines, here's a sample grocery shopping list:

Chicken or turkey breast

Fish (e.g., salmon, trout, cod)

Tofu

Low-fiber vegetables (e.g., green beans, carrots, spinach)

Low-fiber fruits (e.g., bananas, melons, peaches)

Whole grain pasta or bread

Brown rice

Quinoa

Beans and lentils

Low-fat dairy products (e.g., skim milk, low-fat yogurt, reduced-fat cheese)

Olive oil or canola oil

Herbs and spices for seasoning (e.g., garlic, basil, oregano)

Remember to read food labels carefully to check for hidden sources of fat, and try to limit your intake of sugar and salt as well. With a little planning and preparation, you can create healthy, delicious meals that are gentle on your pancreas and support your overall health and well-being.

C. Meal Planning Tips and Tricks

Choose low-fat proteins: When selecting proteins, choose lean options such as chicken, turkey, fish, and legumes. Avoid fatty meats like beef, pork, and lamb as they can trigger pancreatitis symptoms.

Avoid processed foods: Processed foods like fast foods, packaged snacks, and ready-to-eat meals are high in fat, sugar, and salt which can cause inflammation and exacerbate pancreatitis symptoms. Opt for fresh, whole foods instead.

Increase fiber intake: Incorporate fiber-rich foods like fruits, vegetables, whole grains, and legumes in your meal plan. Fiber can help regulate digestion and prevent constipation which can worsen pancreatitis symptoms.

Avoid alcohol: Alcohol consumption can cause inflammation and damage to the pancreas. It's best to avoid alcohol completely if you have pancreatitis.

Choose low-fat cooking methods: When cooking, choose low-fat methods like baking, grilling, roasting, steaming, and boiling. Avoid frying or sautéing foods in oil as it can increase fat content and trigger symptoms.

Limit sugar intake: High sugar intake can cause inflammation and affect blood sugar levels which can be harmful for people with pancreatitis. Avoid sugary drinks, desserts, and processed snacks.

Incorporate anti-inflammatory foods: Foods like ginger, turmeric, salmon, olive oil, nuts, and seeds have anti-inflammatory properties that can help reduce inflammation and alleviate pancreatitis symptoms.

Consult with a registered dietitian: Consulting with a registered dietitian can be helpful in creating a personalized meal plan that suits your nutritional needs and preferences while managing pancreatitis symptoms.

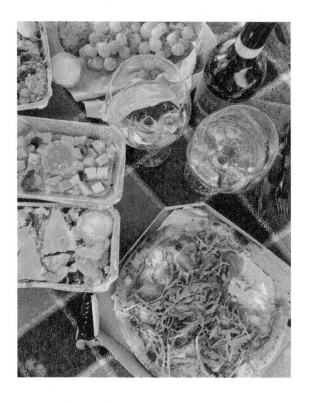

2 Anti Inflammatory Food

CHAPTER 4

Bonus Resources

Grocery list: A detailed list of ingredients needed to prepare all the meals included in the meal plan, making it easier to shop for and ensure you have all the necessary items.

Meal prep guide: A step-by-step guide on how to prepare the meals in the meal plan efficiently, including tips on batch cooking and storage.

Recipe modifications: Tips on how to modify recipes to meet your individual needs, such as reducing fat content, adjusting portion sizes, or swapping out certain ingredients.

Nutritional information: A breakdown of the nutritional content of each recipe, including calorie, fat, protein, and carbohydrate counts, to help you track your intake and make informed choices.

Food diary: Printable templates to track what you eat each day, which can help you identify triggers and monitor your progress.

Pancreatitis education: Educational resources on what pancreatitis is, how to manage it, and the role of diet in the management of pancreatitis.

Community support: Access to an online community of people with pancreatitis or other related conditions, where you can share experiences, get support, and find additional resources.

It's important to note that the specific bonus resources included in a pancreatitis cookbook meal plan may vary depending on the author or publisher.

A. Pancreatitis-Friendly Ingredients Guide

Low-fat proteins: Lean meats such as chicken, turkey, fish, and tofu are good options for people with pancreatitis. Avoid high-fat meats like beef, pork, and lamb.

Low-fat dairy: Non-fat or low-fat dairy products like skim milk, low-fat yogurt, and low-fat cheese are better choices for people with pancreatitis. Avoid dairy products with added fat.

Whole grains: Whole grains such as brown rice, whole wheat bread, and oatmeal are good options for people with pancreatitis. Avoid refined grains like white bread and pasta.

Fruits and vegetables: Fruits and vegetables are an important part of any diet, but people with pancreatitis should choose low-acidic fruits such as apples, bananas, and pears. Avoid high-acidic fruits like oranges, lemons, and tomatoes. Cooked or canned vegetables are better than raw vegetables as they are easier to digest.

Healthy fats: Small amounts of healthy fats like olive oil, avocado, and nuts are okay for people with pancreatitis. However, people with pancreatitis should avoid high-fat foods like fried foods and processed snacks.

Spices and herbs: Spices and herbs can add flavor to meals without adding excess fat or sugar. However, people with pancreatitis should avoid spicy or highly seasoned foods as they can irritate the pancreas.

Fluids: Staying hydrated is important for people with pancreatitis. Drinking plenty of water and other clear fluids like herbal tea or low-sugar sports drinks can help.

It's important to note that everyone's experience with pancreatitis is different, and some foods that are okay for one person may not be okay for another. It's best to consult with a healthcare provider or registered dietitian to create a personalized meal plan that works for you.

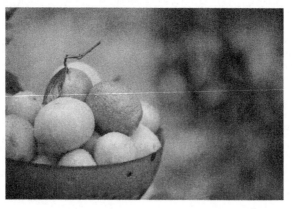

B. Frequently Asked Questions (FAQs)

What is pancreatitis?

Pancreatitis is an inflammation of the pancreas, an organ below the stomach that makes hormones that control blood sugar levels and digesting enzymes.

Why does pancreatitis occur?

Pancreatitis can be caused by several factors, including alcohol abuse, gallstones, high levels of triglycerides in the blood, certain medications, infections, and autoimmune disorders.

What pancreatitis signs and symptoms are there?

The symptoms of pancreatitis include severe pain in the upper abdomen, nausea and vomiting, fever, rapid heartbeat, and a swollen and tender abdomen.

What are the dietary recommendations for pancreatitis?

The dietary recommendations for pancreatitis include avoiding alcohol, reducing fat intake, eating small, frequent meals, avoiding spicy and high-fiber foods, and staying well-hydrated.

What is the purpose of a pancreatitis cookbook meal plan?

The purpose of a pancreatitis cookbook meal plan is to provide individuals with pancreatitis with nutritious, flavorful, and easy-to-prepare meal options that are tailored to their specific dietary needs and restrictions.

What are some examples of foods that should be included in a pancreatitis cookbook meal plan?

Some examples of foods that should be included in a pancreatitis cookbook meal plan include lean proteins such as chicken, fish, and turkey; low-fat dairy products such as yogurt and skim milk; complex carbohydrates such as whole grains, fruits, and vegetables; and healthy fats such as olive oil and avocados.

Are there any foods that should be avoided in a pancreatitis cookbook meal plan?

Yes, there are certain foods that should be avoided in a pancreatitis cookbook meal plan, including alcohol, fatty and fried foods, spicy foods, high-fiber foods, and processed foods.

Can a pancreatitis cookbook meal plan be customized to individual preferences and dietary restrictions?

Yes, a pancreatitis cookbook meal plan can be customized to individual preferences and dietary restrictions, such as vegetarian or gluten-free diets.

What are some tips for following a pancreatitis cookbook meal plan?

Some tips for following a pancreatitis cookbook meal plan include planning ahead, reading food labels carefully, cooking with healthy fats and low-fat cooking methods, and staying well-hydrated.

Is it important to consult with a healthcare professional before starting a pancreatitis cookbook meal plan?

Yes, it is important to consult with a healthcare professional before starting a pancreatitis cookbook meal plan, as they can provide individualized dietary recommendations and monitor progress.

C. Tools and Equipment

Recommended

When it comes to cooking and meal planning for pancreatitis, there are several tools and equipment that can make the process easier and more efficient.

Here are some recommendations:

Non-stick cookware: Non-stick cookware is essential for cooking low-fat meals for pancreatitis. This type of cookware helps prevent food from sticking to the surface, which can be especially helpful when cooking with limited amounts of oil.

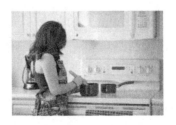

Food processor or blender: A food processor or blender is useful for pureeing or blending foods to create smooth and easy-to-digest meals. These appliances can also be used to chop vegetables or make sauces and dips.

Steamer basket: Steaming is a great way to cook vegetables and fish without adding fat or oil. A steamer basket can be used on top of a pot of boiling water to gently cook foods and preserve their nutrients.

Digital kitchen scale: A digital kitchen scale can help you accurately measure portion sizes and ingredients. This is especially important when following a pancreatitis meal plan that requires specific measurements.

Oven-safe baking dish: An oven-safe baking dish can be used to bake low-fat meals, such as baked chicken or fish. Look for a dish that is large enough to hold your meal without overcrowding it.

Instant-read thermometer: An instant-read thermometer can help you ensure that meats are cooked to the proper temperature without overcooking them. This is especially important for people with pancreatitis, as overcooked meats can be difficult to digest.

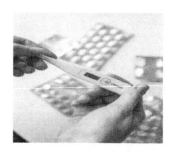

Vegetable peeler: A vegetable peeler is essential for peeling and slicing vegetables, which can be a key part of a pancreatitis meal plan.

Sharp knives: Sharp knives are important for cutting and chopping ingredients safely and efficiently. Dull knives can be dangerous and make meal prep more difficult.

By having these tools and equipment in your kitchen, you can make cooking and meal planning for pancreatitis easier and more enjoyable.

CONCLUSION

Pancreatitis is a condition in which the pancreas becomes inflamed and can cause a variety of symptoms such as abdominal pain, nausea, and vomiting. A well-planned diet is an essential part of managing pancreatitis, as certain foods can aggravate the condition and cause further damage to the pancreas.

A pancreatitis cookbook meal plan is an excellent resource for those looking to manage their pancreatitis symptoms through diet. The meal plan should include foods that are low in fat and easy to digest, such as lean proteins, vegetables, and fruits.

When creating a pancreatitis meal plan, it's important to keep in mind that every individual's needs may vary. Some may need more protein, while others may need more carbohydrates. Consulting with a registered dietitian can help ensure that the meal plan is personalized to fit the individual's needs.

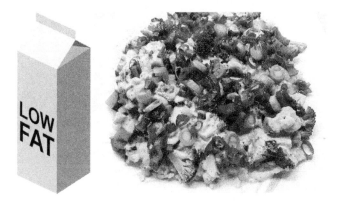

The cookbook meal plan can be a valuable tool for managing pancreatitis symptoms. It should include low-fat, easy-to-digest foods and be personalized to meet the individual's unique needs. By following a well-planned meal plan, individuals with pancreatitis can improve their quality of life and reduce the risk of further damage to the pancreas.